A Life
Depends On It

A Life Depends On It

A Self-defense Primer for Teachers,
Parents, and Students

Edward DeMedeiros

Library of Congress Control Number:		2014905473
ISBN:	Hardcover	978-1-4931-8877-2
	Softcover	978-1-4931-8878-9
	eBook	978-1-4931-8879-6

This book was printed in the United States of America.

Rev. date: 03/19/2014

To order additional copies of this book, contact:
Xlibris LLC
1-888-795-4274
www.Xlibris.com
Orders@Xlibris.com
616239

INDEX

EVERYTHING
IS SELF-DEFENSE

This book is not your typical *how-to* book, although it does have some how-to in it—it won't teach you any one thing that is mysterious or *secret*; we will leave that to books designed for that purpose. This book is meant to take you beyond kicking and punching to the realities of having punched or kicked, to dealing with bullies, the law, women's self-protection, and the attendant realities missing from so many martial arts schools and family conversations. And yes, we'll address some techniques, too, but more toward the necessity of doing things correctly as opposed to the specifics of the techniques in and of themselves. This book addresses some very fundamental questions, such as, "Why did my child—a gifted athlete—get beat up?" or "Why are many *women only* self-defense seminars impractical?" and "How can I bully-proof my child?" This book is *our* conversation on how to learn and better understand martial arts and self-defense.

From the moment we wake up to the moment we bolt our doors and crawl back into bed we have had a full day of self-defense. We brush our teeth to defend against tooth decay, we dress to protect ourselves from the elements, we look both ways when crossing the street, we drive cautiously to avoid accidents, we attend school so that we may learn how the world works and not be cheated, we go to work to protect ourselves from homelessness, and even amusement rides have seat-belts. Everything really is self-defense. We learn to read critically, we learn how to apply mathematics to our financial affairs, we learn the basics of law, politics, history and current trends of the society and the world we live in AND we learn to kick and punch. All these things help us make our way in the world, and can be seen as self-defense of or from one thing or another. It may not be a constant, worrisome, or paranoid self-defense, but we do it—it is how we survive.

Looked at from the point of view that *everything is self-defense* we can begin to grasp the enormous roll self-defense plays in our lives. When once we may have thought protecting ourselves entailed knowing how to escape a madman's clutches, we now find we use self-defense everywhere we go.

AUTHOR'S INTENTIONS

As a novice martial arts student I had felt that there were fundamental pieces of the martial arts and self-defense puzzle missing—perhaps having started my formal training as an adult gave me a unique perspective; I had already lived through many altercations while growing up, and had come to meet a wide variety of people from all walks of life. I felt that people could get hurt because of an inflated or misguided sense of ability, ego, pride, or accomplishment; attitudes which may lead many unsuspecting martial arts students to fail at the very task martial arts were designed to overcome. During my years of study I've heard parents complain how their children, ranking students and gifted athletes in the practice studio, were beaten up and humiliated in the real world that exists away from the practice hall. I did not know, as a student, that it was not just a small piece of the puzzle that was missing from martial arts training, but that there were huge differences between what goes on in the martial arts studio and what it takes to overcome physical and mental challenges presented by others.

My goal, my intention, is to help people become aware of some of the facts and fallacies that pervade martial arts and self-defense. Everything contained herein has been taught to my students and to my children and to my grandchildren. It is hoped that the lessons, anecdotes, and ideas presented here will help prospective students, parents, and martial arts instructors revisit what they believe martial arts to be and how it is taught and can be taught regarding self-defense in the real world.

I hope this book will elicit a conversation among teachers and their students and between parents and their children—whether in the martial art schools or homes. I hope it will help start the flow of ideas that can be used to build a successful self-defense program.

I leave it up to parents, students, teachers, as well as the casual reader, to take what they believe to be useful and to exercise caution and restraint when trying any of the ideas, training methods, or techniques contained herein. Talk to an attorney regarding the use of force, as the author is not providing legal advice, but only the author's opinion. Taken to an extreme any idea or technique can become counterproductive, and even harmful. As such, the reader assumes all responsibility for the use, or attempted use, of any information contained in these pages.

"... and though we still hold that a warrior should have more skills and knowledge than only the craft of weapons and slaying, we esteem a warrior, nonetheless, above men of other crafts."

J.R.R Tolkien
"The Two Towers"

"... to leave the world a bit better.
Whether by a healthy child,
A garden patch,
Or a redeemed social condition,
To know even one life has breathed easier because you have lived,
This is to have succeeded."

Ralph Waldo Emerson

This book is dedicated to my children-
Michael, Crystal, and Katie

ONE

WHAT MANY WANT
vs. WHAT MOST GET

I believe most people considering enrollment in a martial arts school, program, or academy do so because they believe they will get useful training to develop skills that will enable them to defend themselves. They want skills that are practical, easy to learn, and immediately useful. And while the words 'practical' and 'useful' can be somewhat vague it is because no two situations are exactly the same, either in intensity, threat level, or number. We enroll in self-defense schools because therein, it is hoped, are answers to the questions of self-preservation. It could be that a child had recurring bad experiences at school or in a park or playground. It could be because a job or a job location brings one into close proximity to areas or neighborhoods one would not ordinarily go to or be in. The reasons are many and varied, but the need is common—the need to learn to be able to protect one's self—and perhaps others from harm or threat of harm.

This sounds straightforward—almost too easy. Well here's where it may not be so easy: It is easy if applied in a straightforward manner in which only self-defense techniques are taught—such as is taught to military personnel—but most schools won't teach straightforward self defense because it is something easily learned, and once learned, students would go about their lives with a minimum of refreshers, if any at all, and may never step into a martial arts school ever again. From a strictly business perspective it would be in the school's best interest to keep the students coming back many, many times. A profitable business model is one in which the information is doled out in bits and pieces over a protracted length of time— which in many cases can be years of instruction. The schools, after all, are in business to make money, and having a steady client base will ensure their longevity, success, and profit.

The crux of learning from a martial arts school is that in order to learn self-defense one must also learn physical fitness; stretching, running, and any number of calisthenics. Students are disciplined to instantly obey every command as if they had joined a military unit. Students are also taught many different blocks, strikes, kicks, evasions, and counter-attacks. We're talking about thousands or even tens of thousands of repetitions of all of the above and all the special stances that go with each technique of the "art." "But wait," as the TV commercials proclaim, "there's more!"

As part of martial arts curriculum there is what is known as 'forms'—often, groups of forms known as 'sets'. Forms are the 'art' part of martial arts. Forms are the choreographed sequences of movements that somewhat resemble dance—it is a string of movements that demonstrate balance, timing, rhythm, and coordination—something useful in the development of graceful and coordinated movement. It is tedious and time-consuming and is very impressive in practice among student peers, and at competitions for trophies and medals. It's what the famous swordsman, Miyamoto Musashi, called the 'flowers' of martial arts, because it bore little or no real usable fruit to self-defense and it's applications in real life—something that is the topic of much debate regarding the benefits of forms, even among the martial arts community. This is not meant to describe all schools that teach forms as flowery or for show. There are those schools in which the practice of forms is the central core of their self-defense training program and art. The forms of many of the grappling arts are practical and immediately useful. Outside of the grappling arts, forms are the training regimen schools spend a great deal of time perfecting and yet it is the thing most quickly forgotten once the student quits the school for any length of time; even a few weeks away from the practice studio will erode the ability to correctly demonstrate forms—if they are not entirely forgotten.

As an aside, here I must say that there are some arts that I consider more practical and immediately useful. Those arts are of the grappling nature, such as, Judo, Jujitsu, and ChiNa, to name a few. And some, like Krav Maga, are of the kickboxing style and are very practical. Boxing also comes to mind—although it doesn't have forms in the conventional sense—neither do the current wave of mixed martial arts schools.

All these things are being said to give you some idea of what is out there and what to expect. If a school that is predominately about teaching forms, or earning trophies seems to be to your liking, I say, "Go for it." You will get some self-defense benefits, but probably over the long term. If immediate and practical self-defense is what you want or need, then perhaps boxing is for you. It is like the old saying: "All roads lead to Rome", but some will take you the long way there.

So, once again, what do we want, and why are we here? We want to learn how to defend ourselves if and when the need arises. We want the training, ideas, and techniques needed to develop the skills necessary to achieve the self-defense goal. And we're here, with this book in hand to get ideas we can use to help us to understand something of what martial arts is in many schools, and what it could be with some new ideas or additions to current training regimens.

Two

DO WE NEED A
MARTIAL ARTS SCHOOL?

You probably do. Martial arts schools have most, if not all, of the equipment and necessary space to practice in—not to mention all your fellow students to practice your technique with and upon and to offer you encouragements.

From a strictly self-defense point of view, it is not necessary to have much equipment with which to practice. Of course if you happen to belong to a military unit, or police or security organization that works with weapons of any kind, you would need the appropriate weapons and equipment to train with. For example, people who work in the security services may need to know how to disarm someone who is holding a long or a short gun, or a knife. In that case they need to train with those weapons, and more likely, as civilian, you would not.

Also of importance is the length of time it takes to learn practical self-defense. No two students learn at the same rate, nor do all teachers have the same ability to convey ideas and techniques so that all students can learn what is being taught. It becomes difficult to pin down a time within which one becomes proficient at hands-on, physical self-defense. I believe that if the focus of the program is strictly hands on self-defense a person could become reasonably proficient within a span of three months to one year. Too short, or too long of a time period? Again it depends on the learning abilities verses teaching abilities as well as the number of classes available to students per week or per month, and whether students avail themselves of all classes being offered.

Getting back to the original question at the beginning of this chapter: Do you need a martial arts school? I opened this chapter with the statement, "You probably do." And here at this point in the chapter I'll say, "Maybe not."

I believe you or your child may not need a professionally run school to teach yourself, your child, or a group of friends some practical self-defense. Let's face it, many people are competent readers who can understand directions given in a book, video, or DVD, and translate those directions into physical actions with willing friends and family. There are many gifted and natural teachers who have had little or no training in a field they teach or help teach. There are many parents helping their youngsters learn to catch a ball, swing bat, or swing a tennis racquet; the possibility most certainly exists for a determined person to learn and teach many aspects usually taught in schools, or taught by others. I know of groups of teenaged boys who are doing just that—teaching themselves grappling—and quite successfully, too.

Also, and once-upon-a-time, children were allowed to play and wrestle—it was natures way of training the young in defensive techniques, as well as building endurance, strength, and even peer bonding. Animals of every kind do exactly that! Children who play similar games and who have similar interests and tastes tend to become fast friends.

Play wrestling helps build confidence; it is something children do naturally when allowed to "rough-house" in the park or play ground—except we don't encourage or allow it any more because society is leaning away from the physical arts; it's just not socially acceptable these days. But that doesn't preclude parents from gently wrestling with a very young son or daughter. From about the time a child can crawl the child can play wrestle. I recommend a game of "capture" in which a parent will gently capture the child and let him or her work free. Every time the child crawls away, or works free, the parent could make a surprised and happy show for the child benefit so that the child will be encouraged to play the wrestle game again and again. If it can't be done in the school yard or playground, at least it can be done at home, and it makes for a great bonding experience.

I "play wrestled" with my children from the time they could crawl—I'd fake capturing them and they would squirm their way in one direction or another to make an escape. They loved the game. As they got older I made it more difficult to escape—I held them a bit longer. And in the wrestling matches I had with my son, we would work quite hard to pin or take each other down. By the time he was thirteen and fourteen years of age I was having great difficulty getting him to the floor and more than once he took me down quite hard. After a few landings like that I realized the time had come for us to stop wrestling—he was getting to big and to strong. He didn't need dad's training anymore.

During the entire history of our wrestling experience I never told my children they were learning a martial art—or any art, for that matter. It was simply good parent/child bonding and a healthy activity for us all. They did not grow up to be bullies; as a matter of fact my son's confidence allowed him to be the protector when he saw in justices and bulling at school, and when he entered a structured martial arts environment he quickly became one of the students others looked up to. His confidence, personality, and skill earned him rank and admiration.

Do we need a martial arts school in order to learn self-defense? Maybe yes, you do. Or maybe no, you don't. Yes, if you want to earn ranks (belts) and become certified by the school's parent organization as a black belt—bearing in mind certification does not equal proficiency in self-defense. And, for reasons already given—depending on the art studied—certification could indicate self-defense proficiency. Yes, if you believe the training at a particular school is beneficial, useful, or realistic. Yes, if your goal is to go through the motions of fighting in tournaments so as to win trophies or medals—maybe get your name or your child's name in a local newspaper. Yes, if you are not able or your child is too big to play wrestle with.

No, you can get by if you can't afford professional lessons. There are books, videos, DVDs, and free video instructions available through the internet that will show and explain many self-defense techniques you can learn and share with family and willing friends.

The question of whether we need a martial arts school or not becomes rather academic when actually faced with the reality of self-defense. In the following chapters we examine self-defense options available in the actual practice of self preservation.

THREE

PERMISSIONS

When I was a lower-ranking student parents would come in to the studio with their children wanting to know what went wrong with a recent altercation their child had with another child in the schoolyard. Sometimes the location would be a park, but the questions were always the same: "What went wrong?"

I was surprised when my instructor could not form an answer to their simple question. It is a fundamental failure to parents when their children cannot defend themselves because something happened or failed to happen in the life of this child—this student—to make the children question their ability, and to make the parents question the teacher or process they are paying for. It is a shame when that happens—teachers feel bad, parents feel bad, and students, too,—not knowing if they did anything wrong, or if they should have done something differently—feel bad.

We want our children to succeed in all the areas we send them to be trained in. We send them to public or private schools so that they will be able to pass exams and use their knowledge in the world outside. We expect no less from martial arts schools and academies. If something is not working, then perhaps the problem or problems need to be revisited. Perhaps the answer can be found in two parts—actually there are many more components that make for a complete understanding, but we will address two of them now and more as we progress through the remaining chapters.

The first part may be the most obvious: Is the art suitable or suited to the student? In other words, is the student comfortable and proficient in the art being studied? Is the training realistic and viable to today's modes of social interaction? Many schools are teaching 'old world' and old styles of martial arts that have elements in practice that were only used decades, or centuries ago. Some rituals being taught make no sense today—I have never been to a tea ceremony, or any other ceremony or dinner, where I had to sit on my feet and walk about on my knees, and perhaps practice drawing my sword from that position—so why would I, or anyone other than history buff, need to learn to do so when all we want is hands-on self-defense? Also, is the school focusing much of the student's effort and energy toward tournament proficiency to the neglect of practical self-defense? We touched on this subject earlier regarding "forms", so here we will focus on tournament sparring.

Sparring at tournaments, and in the studio, is not the same as fighting for self-defense or survival. Sparring is a rules-oriented form of fighting wherein punching to the face is not allowed during competition. Other sparring rules state that no kicks are allowed to the opponent's legs, and that no kicks or strikes are allowed beyond the natural line of the arms—back, kidneys, back of the head, or spine. Oddly enough kicks are allowed to the head on the theory that opponents should see the leg long before it strikes due to the distance it must travel. So far we have a limited number of techniques available when training for and engaging in tournament or school sparring. But that's not all.

No one who enters a sparring match—especially at competition—is allowed to participate unless they are wearing the appropriate and necessary protective equipment. Competitors must wear padded foam head, leg, foot, chest, and groin protection, as well as mouth guards. Women are required to wear protection, too. These are necessary, not only to protect the student/competitor, but to help eliminate injuries both physical and legal. Most students will train in their respective studios with equipment on so as to be thoroughly comfortable with it in the studio and the competition arena. What all this equipment does not protect anyone from is the reality that exists outside of the studio or competition arena where no one is wearing foam, and when, in all probability, it would do the most good.

Secondly, students need permission to actively defend themselves.

It would seem like something that would go without saying that receiving permission to defend one's self would be fundamental in the study of any martial art—we tend to intuit that it is, like something implied in the very nature of the study. It is almost as implied that all martial artists are 'tough, kick-butt' people. Well, at least the potential is there even if the training and permissions are not.

I believe that students should have permission from the teacher to defend themselves. I believe permission should be given within sight and hearing of the parents, and that the parents should be encouraged to give their permission, as well. Parents and children should be encouraged to enter into a dialog that relieves the child of any confusion regarding self-protection. My question to parents has often been, "Do you want to pick your child up from the principal's office or police station, or do you want to pick him up from the hospital or morgue?" Your child, my student, needs to know if and when it is okay to defend himself, and needs your okay to do so. To send a child to school with the admonition, "Okay, honey, have a nice day. Don't get into any trouble," leaves the child very few options during a personal emergency. Have you ever received an admonition such as that? Did it give you any reassurance or indication of what or how you were to proceed in any given situation? If you put yourself in the child or students place you can see how important it is to have the information or permission.

It is the lack of real-world training and scenario/role-playing that will cause failure at attempted self-defense. It is also because we have failed to give our children permission to act as their own protectors. In the end it becomes our failure as teachers and parents. And that, my friends, is the answer my teacher could not articulate, and why children get beat up even when they have the talent to avoid, or end, an attack or confrontation when they are otherwise physically able to do so.

FOUR

SO MUCH EQUIPMENT!

The first day at a martial arts school may include instructions of this nature, "Okay, the first thing we do here is we take off our shoes; we never want to walk on the mats with shoes on. And, oh yah, never kick the heavy bag, or anything else in here, with your shoes on, okay? Also, you're going to need protective head, chest, hand, shin, and foot gear. We sell all that stuff at the desk out front. Get yourself a groin cup, too. Uniforms will be in next week, so wear sweatpants until then."

Within a short time of enrolling we find ourselves barefoot and covered in ten pieces of foam protective gear and wearing a groin cup. What's wrong with this picture from the self-defense standpoint? It is incongruous with what we would be wearing the other twenty-three hours of the day, and it certainly would not be what we would be wearing in a mall parking lot, school cafeteria, or city park.

While I do agree a certain amount of protection is very good in the early learning stages, I do wonder why we continue to use them long after a student has demonstrated proficiency, control, and skill in sparring (an activity resembling the game of "Tag", but with gloves on). Let's not forget what all the sparring is training for. We can never assume all students will ever do in their lives is spar—as if fighting for survival will never happen.

Training in bare feet is not for the benefit of the student, it is for the protection of the floor mats. And while teachers say training in bare feet toughens the feet, how often, with the exception of a summer's day at the beach, are we walking around barefoot? By protecting floor mats, teachers deprive students the opportunity to know what it feels like to spar, or fight, in shoes—something that could easily unbalance (mentally or physically) a student unaccustomed to fighting in shoes. Small things do make a difference.

To illustrate my point I offer this true story about detrimental training methods: A certain police force trained recruits to retrieve their spent gun cartridges from the floor during training, and to 'pocket' the spent brass as a way to clean up after themselves. The officers did this every time they trained and when one day some of them were involved in a real fire-fight with real bad-guys, some of them were shot because they bent down to retrieve spent brass. They did what they were trained to do, and it cost them.

Another spurious piece of martial arts equipment is uniforms. Martial arts uniforms are a throwback to peasant garb of bygone years; they are spacious and allow plenty of room for movements like punching, kicking, and stretching. Again, like protective gear, they will not be wearing this uniform outside of the training area. Everyday clothing is more restrictive; they have a very different feel, and, like shoes, that unaccustomed feel could unbalance a well rehearsed technique.

The proposition I make here is simple yet practical: Periodically have the students train in and with whatever they have on. If they come to the studio wearing winter gloves, for example, have them work on their techniques with their gloves on. Try the same regarding boots, shoes, shorts, sweatshirts, and even coats. These changes in training apparel will change the sparring and self-defense dynamic, but it will lend authenticity to what is being learned. Remember what happened to those police officers because someone was preoccupied with keeping their shooting range clear of brass casings. While the "range" may have been kept clear, the officers suffered needlessly. Poor training has consequences. Don't let this happen to your children or your students.

FIVE

IS WHAT WE ARE
LEARNING EFFECTIVE?

Depictions of self-defense techniques in martial arts books, and in many studios, is woefully lacking in realism. Open a self-defense book and there will be many examples of self-rescue techniques. Watch or attend a self-defense seminar and you will be exposed to techniques that are supposed to work. All we have, whether book or studio training, is nothing more than an academic exercise—it's supposed to work, so we assume it will.

Let's use a two-handed choke to a "victim's" throat as an example. Books, and many schools, teach choke self-rescue techniques that have the aggressor's hands on the 'victim's shoulders or close to the neck, but never actually grabbing the neck. The victim then does the appropriate and approved technique, and everyone is happy because the technique worked. Or did it?

Absent realism—or a modicum of reality—can lead one to a false sense of accomplishment and security, believing one is actually good at something when in fact they are not. Missing from this training scenario was the anger, the pushing or pulling, the surprise, the fear, the name-calling/swearing, or intent to harm. It begs the question: How are we going to react when those external elements happen in real life?

Of course we can't include all aspects of a violent encounter, but we can make each technique a bit harder to escape from. The choke in our example can actually be applied to the neck and throat with a mild or moderate pressure, and the "victim" can be forced to move backward by the aggressor's action of pushing the victim. Couple that with verbal threats and taunts and we have a much more dynamic and realistic scenario from which the victim must escape, or escape and counter-attack.

In the case of wrist grabbing escapes, have the attacker pull the victim as one would an attempted kidnapping. Use your imagination to create plausible attack scenarios and your level of teaching or learning will increase dramatically. Above all don't get so carried away with the "reality" aspect of the training that you actually hurt someone. Remember, everyone wants to go home at the end of the training session, not to the emergency room of the local hospital.

Work on these training ideas and techniques with caution. This principle applies to headlocks, wrist grabs, and just about any self-defense technique one is trying to impart to the student. The point here is: it is fine to start the training session in a static, hands-on-shoulders training style, but before the day is out there should be some realism added to the training. In this way, what the student learns today becomes immediately useful. This is the same way professionals train, whether bodyguards, Secret Service, local police departments, or military units. Only by training in a realistic fashion can we expect to have success using self-defense. Barry's (not his real name) story will help illustrate the point.

Barry was an 18 year old, 5'10" and 155 pound "nice guy, next-door neighbor" type of young man we see walking the campuses every day, and he had come to us to learn the art of kickboxing—or more realistically "white collar" kickboxing like you see on the infomercials on television exercise programs. He was quiet and humble and eager to learn. He absorbed every technique like one who was born to be a kick-boxer; his stances and movements were smooth, his stamina was impressive, his technique flawless. Seldom did he miss his training appointments and he did everything he was told to do. Like most young men he was very eager to spar, so we eventually decided to let him try boxing a real opponent.

But Barry had a problem—one that is at the heart of this book—in that everything he had learned was "supposed to work." It was academic—like reading a book on how to fly an airplane and then trying to fly the real thing. So when he faced his first opponent—his trial-by-fire—he was unable to do the things he could do so well when no one was facing him and trying to hit him. He ran around the ring with his gloved hands covering his head; he had never faced anyone who— even without anger—was ready, willing, and able to hit him.

Barry did not enter the ring for some time after his first attempt; we had to train him in a way that was more realistic and desensitizing so that his fear of being hurt was turned in to a comfortable familiarity. His original problem did not stem from inability—he had the physical tools—it's because he had never had a fight in his life in or out of the schoolyard, park, or street. As a child he had never been spanked nor wrestled with his parents or friends. In short, his mental fear of being hit or hurt terrified him and he froze.

Barry's situation is not unique. There are large numbers of youngsters and adults who think they can fight because they can get "mad enough". Yet when it comes right down to it they may be confusing anger and willingness for ability.

There are three elements necessary to make one a better fighter or increases our self-defense skill level. The first is WILLINGNESS. It sounds so simple, but we need to recognize who we are and who we want our young people or our own children to become—it's a personal philosophy of life, and something that should also be discussed at home or in the studio. There are two basic types of people when it comes to self-defense. There are "peaceful" people and there are "pacifists". The peaceful person goes about life wishing no harm and doing no harm but will defend him or herself if given no other option. A pacifist, too, goes about life doing no harm and wishing no harm, but will not hurt anyone under any circumstances—hoping instead the attacker does not hurt him too much—or kill him—and that the attack is over soon. It is important we recognize who we or our children are so that we can afford them ideas and techniques for self-preservation. Are we willing to defend ourselves?

Next we need ABILITY. Ability is where the physical training enters the self-defense equation. Without knowing how to punch, or kick, for example, we will fall short on our defense if we are attacked.

It will not be of much help if we are angry or determined if we cannot do "something" to ward off the attack. This is also why we send our children off to learn martial arts or boxing while they are young—so they will have the ability to take care of themselves for their entire lives.

READINESS is the third part of our self-defense equation. It is the combination of self-defense theory (like reading the book on how to fly an airplane), plus knowledge of the physical art (making us able to defend), coupled with as much "realistic" training as possible. If the training is not realistic, then what we have is a weak imitation of self-defense, and one is not considered to be "ready".

Barry eventually did learn to fight. He learned to face his fears and his opponents. He was able to do so because we included physical contact while he was working on his techniques or hitting the heavy-bag. If I was holding the hand-mitts, I would hit him gently on the head, sides, or stomach. As he progressed, I was able to strike him harder, even adding verbal taunts and challenges. It didn't take long for him to be able to "suck-it-up" and become a formidable fighter—one his sparring partners could respect in the ring.

It doesn't matter if one trains in a martial arts studio, at home with mom and dad, or horseplay with friends, what matters in training is the modicum of realism that will keep us from freezing up at a critical moment because of an unfamiliarity with what is happening around us or to us. What matters more than belt ranking in a martial art school is the willingness, readiness, and ability realism can bring to any self-defense training regimen.

Six

THERE ARE MANY BULLIES AMONG US

Much is being brought to light regarding bullying; almost every month the news media reports young people being victimized (abused) in one way or another by other young people. Sometimes the bullying is so traumatizing it prompts the victim to suicide. Yet bullying has been with us as long as humans have existed—it's part of human nature. It doesn't matter what name we put to it—children abusing children (bullying), adults bullying children (child abuse), adults bullying adults (assault), children bullying parents (parental abuse)—it happens every day. And even though there are laws being enacted to help curb bullying, laws won't stop bullying any more than laws have stopped rape, murder, or littering. All types of crime continue, and so will bullying. Dealing with physical bullying is a self-defense problem, and one that students can learn to recognize and stop.

There is also what can only be perceived as verbal bullying. I say perceived because in many instances the term bullying is misapplied and is not an intentional, intensive, or consistent event.

It is the rare child who has learned the art of diplomacy . . . a child who will couch the things they say in filtered terms or descriptions. Young people often say exactly what is on their mind—often very unfiltered and undiplomatically. If they see what they think is odd . . . wrongly or otherwise . . . they are apt to say what they think in a blunt and straight forward fashion. The object of their ridicule may be someone's shoes, clothing, hair, speech, weight, or choice of socks . . . just about anything may be the subject of unfiltered observation. If a child's choice of dress, for example, is so different from his peers he may find those same peers collectively chastising him for not being a member of the group.

It's almost something tribal that happens . . . either the child starts wearing what the others wear or he must continue suffering for his differences. While this may be uncomfortable for the child, and a source of worry for his parents, it is identical to what happens in many groups and packs in nature; an animal that is ill, shows behavior or demeanor different than the pack is often rejected or set upon by the members of the group. While we may be at the top of the food chain we are never above nature, and, as stated above, laws will not change bullying . . . even if the law tries to bully people to change.

When I was a young boy the prevailing wisdom and advice was to punch the offending bully on the nose. It was assumed by parents—well intentioned as they may have been—that punching the bully was the correct option. It is an option, but it shouldn't have to be the only one.

Long before physical bullying begins there is a period of belittlement when the aggressor is testing his intended victim for signs of weakness. The teasing and testing often start as small remarks or small 'put downs'; something the bully can retreat from if the intended victim should prove mentally or physically stronger than himself. The usual retreating remark is, "I was just kidding", or "I wasn't talking about you", or remarks of this nature. I call this the 'interview' stage, and it is the stage we need to recognize and make our students aware of. This is when students need to make their immediate stand.

I suggest to parents and martial arts teachers that there is a way to better "bully—proof" a child, and while it is not guaranteed to work 100% of the time, my children and grandchildren, as well as students, have had great success with the following training techniques.

In my classes I have individual students stand before me and respond to variety of verbal assaults and accusations. We start with simple accusations such as, "You took my pencils from my desk!" Or I may say, "You took my bike and broke it!" Or, "You took my back-pack and threw it in the mud!" ". . . tore my homework!", ". . . stole my toy!", or whatever comes to mind. I then watch the student's reaction and body language, as well as listen to their verbal responses, if there are any. It's amazing to see youngsters fold their arms, or cross their legs, or stare at the floor; they are not yet aware that they can stand up to false accusations and they don't know how to respond. The intention of this exercise is teach students to stand their ground, to look the questioner in the eyes, to stand erect and comfortably with legs apart, and placing their hands on their hips to appear larger. By doing so they project a strong, confident demeanor bullies can shy away from. I often ask them to think of how their mother or father looks when they are displeased, and to use the "look" that says, "I've had enough of this nonsense."

After going through the body language exercise, we work on strong, controlled answers, such as, "I don't know what you're talking about; go ask someone else." or "No, I didn't touch your backpack; ask someone else." The idea is to teach children to form an answer that does not indicate fear of the interviewer (potential bully) and yet is strong, honest, and direct, leaving no room for debate. The "strong voice" can also include yelling, if the student feels the need to do so.

Students should also be made aware that other children sometimes claim skills they don't actually possess, or they may make hand or foot gestures resembling karate movements they've seen in movies, television, or video games. Bullies want others to believe they have power and control. It is important to tell students that it is highly improbable someone their age has had sufficient training and developed enough skill to do the things they claim they can. And while it is possible for anyone, trained or untrained, to hurt someone, it is in all probability they (my students)—perhaps your child—who has the training and skill bullies never suspect.

Very often children will call each other names or make fun of someone's body or clothing. This, too, is bullying and part of the interview process by which bullies measure or 'size up' potential targets to pick on. To help us counter the effects of name calling, we play a "name calling game." The object of this game is to avoid becoming flustered or angry, and to recognize name calling doesn't physically or mentally hurt if we don't let it. It is a form of desensitization and it is fun to do in the studio or home. Use whatever comes to mind, but bear in mind we are dealing with children, so I'd recommend saying, "You've got a pie face."; "You've got a baggy butt!" or "You've got a balloon head!" These are not very threatening taunts, and the children seem to respond positively to them. They may respond, "And the problem is?"; "Yah, I have a big head. It's because I have a large brain."

The point herein is to make students, parents, and teachers aware they have alternatives to the simplistic "punch him in the nose" advice. Appearing confident, not getting flustered, showing a strong, confident demeanor, and using a clear, calm voice works. It has worked for my children and students. Try to remember each student is unique and should be taught techniques and responses suitable to what they tell you—if they tell you—is happening in their neighborhood or school.

Along with bully-proof training should be the admonition that they in turn should not become bullies, and that there is still the need to be kind and courteous to all people, regardless of age. Until they sense someone is trying to intimidate or hurt them in any way there is no need to be hurtful to others.

There is one more thing I believe needs to be mentioned here. Whenever we perceive an encounter as bullying, it is important for us, as adults, not to brush it off as a "kid's thing." The problems faced by youngsters are very real to them, and without proper guidance or mental help too many aspects of their lives can deteriorate. School work can suffer, social interactions may decrease, emotional problems can occur. Outbursts and even introverted behavior can be symptoms of bullying. As adults, we have a responsibility to be on the lookout for things that may be the cause of a change in behavior in the children we are familiar with. If a child will not open up to you, the child may open up to a mental health professional. Never be so busy or embarrassed to ask for help. A life depends on it.

SEVEN

SELF-DEFENSE and the LAW

Self-defense is not simply the execution of punches and kicks brought on by an attack; self-defense has its unique issues regarding the law, as well.

Most of us have heard the statement, "Don't take the law into your own hands." This means that if there is some other way of removing ourselves from a dangerous situation we should, and we should call the police or proper authorities if we can to report the assault, crime, or damage. What we are not supposed to do is act as a judge and dispense punishment, even if someone attacked us.

Nowhere does it say that you cannot defend yourself. Of course you can! It means that once the attacker is stopped from harming you, or the threat is passed, you cannot continue to hit or hurt, nor punish in anyway someone who is no longer a threat to you. Once you are no longer in any danger, you must stop. For example: You have successfully defended yourself from mugger and have knocked him to the ground. Let's further assume he is no longer a threat to you and perhaps has indicated surrender. Under the law, you cannot continue to hit or hurt this person simply because you are angry and want to punish him for his attempt to rob you. If he is retreating you must let him do so. If he is badly injured you may wish to call for medical assistance. In either case, the police should be called and a report made of the incident—this person may be wanted for similar crimes. To harm someone who is no longer a threat to you can get you arrested for assault or battery or both—something that can later lead to a criminal or civil suit against you.

You must comply with all requests made by police once they arrive on the scene. You may be asked to sit in the police car, or on the street curb, or to stand apart from the other person while they try to figure out what happened, and by whom. Keep in mind that the police don't know what happened—they don't know who the attacker was nor who was the victim. Perhaps all they saw when they arrived was you standing over someone and surmise *you* as the attacker.

One way to allay police suspicion of you is to identify yourself right away by saying, "Officer, my name is . . . . I'm a bank-teller (or whatever you do for a living), and this person tried to rob me (or whatever he tried to do)." By identifying yourself to police you immediately begin to demonstrate cooperation and by doing so you may be treated with greater respect than you would have had you left the police to try to sort things on their own.

Also of concern is the possibility of injury you may have sustained during the period of assault or confrontation. Quite often we may be injured and not even know it. As soon as the police or other help arrive ask to be sent to the hospital to be checked out by medical professionals. If you have been struck (punched or kicked) in any way, as for medical assistance.

If you feel that you are being roughly handled by police—if you feel they are antagonistic or unsympathetic to your situation—ask if you should call a lawyer. If you are told that it is probably best to have an attorney present, or especially if they tell you that you are under arrest, say nothing except to identify yourself and that you reserve answering any questions until an attorney is present. Be polite, calm, and firm at all times when dealing with police officers; they were not there when the attack or altercation started and have no way to know what happened until all the facts are made know to them. Remember, "Yes, sir/officer.", or "No, sir/officer." And, "I'm not trying to be rude, sir, but I need to wait for my lawyer's advice before I say anything else." Hopefully you have a lawyer's number handy when you need it.

Children should be given special consideration by adults regarding self-defense, but all too often, and because of zero tolerance school policies, children find that they also have to defend themselves, often alone, against unsympathetic school department personnel. It's as if they are being bullied once again, except this time it's by the adults around them. I'm calling them bullies because of incidents where children as young as 8 and 9 years old were forced to sign papers stating they were aware of school policy regarding "fighting" and are admitting breaking that policy. Administration officials can then point to that paper to justify their actions (further bullying) against the child by meting out its punishment, such as: failing the child for a whole day's work, detention, suspension, or even expulsion—all without any legal or parental representation.

Teachers and administrators often treat children as non-citizens, often opening and checking a student's locker and checking that student's possessions. They have opened and gone through student's backpacks and pockets. School authorities justify these actions (suspension of rights) under the supposed argument that once the student is on school property or within school walls, students and parents abrogate their rights to the school and its administrators—as if children entered a separate country exempt from the laws of the land in the name of unity, safety, and security. From a self-defense standpoint, all adults—teachers and administrators—should be regarded as "strangers" (someone we will define more clearly later) by parents and their children. Remember, the 'school' is much more interested in protecting itself and perpetuating its policies and agendas than they are in protecting your child—regardless of administration claims to the contrary.

In dealing with school authorities it may be advisable to instruct children not to sign anything that is not a classroom assignment and to never admit that they were in a fight. I'd rather have my child say they were "trying to push (the person) who was trying to hit me away." I would further advise children to repeatedly say, "I want you to call my mother (or father).", and to make a fuss about that. Again, they are to sign nothing, and they are to ask that a parent be called. These things, too, should be practiced at home and in the self-defense studios.

As regards studio practice, we must remember that martial arts were developed for things "martial"—things pertaining to war and the military. Many, if not most, of the techniques taught in martial arts schools today simply will not be acceptable in a civilian setting. Unless we now have a kinder, gentler military, techniques taught to soldiers were based on "threat elimination". In other words, if something or someone can possibly be a threat it was "eliminated". As civilians we are to use "threat avoidance" as a primary way to self-protection. We are to use physical violence as a last resort, and we are to do so causing the least amount of damage that is possible and reasonable to use. We cannot strike someone in the throat, for example, and kill them because they simply grabbed our arm. The response in this case would not be justified by the threat. Temper all training so that a more reasonable response is available to different threats. A "one size fits all" regimen of training can lead to all sorts of legal trouble.

This chapter simply cannot cover all of the intricacies regarding the law and self-defense. Its intention is to make martial arts and self-defense teachers, parents, and students aware that there is much more to self-defense than mere punching and kicking. Simple advice, such as, "Punch him in the nose!", or "Kick him in the groin, honey!" will not be adequate. We must realize that if we are ever forced to defend ourselves through physical force we may also end up having to defend ourselves in a court of law or before a school board. It is therefore extremely important for any parent, whether your child is a student of self-defense or not, to speak with a legal professional regarding local and state laws pertaining to self-defense on the street and in the school.

EIGHT

AWARENESS

To be 'aware' is to be informed and conscious.

Much of this book is dedicated to exactly that end; to inform and help teachers, parents, and students become aware and conscious of how much more there is to self-defense than simply punching and kicking, or being able to physically remove someone's hands from us. Self-defense starts with situational awareness—the knowing, seeing, and paying attention that will keep us out of harm's way to begin with. It is nothing more than the same type of situational awareness we learned when we were taught to cross the street—and yes that, too, is self-defense. It may be self-defense against a car, but it is self-defense nonetheless, and probably the first defense lesson any of us can remember.

If we need to look before crossing, wouldn't it make sense to look around when we exit a mall or department store door, or when we leave our homes every morning, or when we cross a parking lot to get to our cars? Of course it does. Many have been abducted or robbed because they failed to do so. Quite often we are so preoccupied with our own thoughts that we simply forget to think beyond our need to get somewhere, often walking with our heads down and keys in hand.

Questions involving situational awareness are typically, "What should we be aware of?", and like our example of street crossing, we should be aware of anything or anyone that does not look like they belong where they are, or anyone who could be a threat to us by their proximity to our property or to ourselves. Anything that seems out of the ordinary should be viewed with suspicion. Any time you have a 'bad feeling' about someone, don't brush it off because you feel you will be impolite; trust your feelings and find a way to remove yourself from their presence, or walk away, walk around, or call for help. There is no shame if you are wrong. It is better to be wrong and hurt someone's feelings than it is to ignore your own feelings and be robbed or killed.

When leaving a department store, for example, it is perfectly okay to ask a store employee to walk you to your vehicle, especially at night (and if they help you with your bags, so much the better).

We are not talking about becoming paranoid and distrusting everyone, because that would be a horrible way to live. What we want to achieve is a greater degree of awareness of whom and of what is around us so that we can react or change what we do in response to that new information.

This advice is applicable to all the places we go, whether it is a restaurant, a theater, a barroom, night club, or library and even a school. And we need to practice "looking" every time we walk through a door to go out from or in to any building. Of course there are places where a greater degree of caution will be needed, such as night clubs, barrooms and anyplace where alcohol is served. If you feel uncomfortable for any reason, if you think there may be violence, if someone is looking at you in an exceptionally long or "hard" manner, then it is probably time for you to leave. Alcohol has different effects on different people, and someone who may start out friendly toward you may soon thereafter be the biggest jerk you know, and you don't have to sit there and take it—get up and leave. It is my belief that people don't do things when drunk that they didn't have the propensity to do before they started drinking. Drinking can be their excuse to release their inner jerk.

Staying alive means staying awake to your surroundings, and staying alert to what is happening around you—just as you would do to cross a street.

NINE

AVOIDANCE AND RECOGNITION

Avoidance, as defined, is: An act or practice of avoiding, departing, or withdrawing from; leave; keep away from; preventing the occurrence or effectiveness.

The above definitions all tell us the same thing—it is the getting away or distancing ourselves from something, or in the case of self-defense, the prevention of having something bad happen to us. Knowing what to avoid is sometimes difficult to say without experience—it is difficult to know, for example, that we must be careful to cross the street. And, like our example, we are taught to cross by those people who have had experience in crossing. Without such experience all one can do—and we do it often—is to admonish our children as they go out the door, "Be careful, honey!" without telling them of what to be careful.

One thing we can be careful of—and this is a very big one as regards self-defense—is our being around loud and aggressive people. It seems they attract much attention, especially in social settings, and it is quite possible their loudness and aggressive point-making can lead to an argument or a physical fight—especially when two or more people are shouting and behaving aggressively toward one another.

This brings us to an ancillary point: People engaged in shouting matches do not seem interested in what the other person is saying, only in what they themselves are saying, and they are trying to block out the other persons point of view. In other words, it's as if they believe that the loudest person "wins". It may have started as a simple discussion, but somehow discussions can devolve into heated and violent arguments.

Avoidance can also mean not getting involved in barroom "politics"—the often alcohol-induced, boisterous, shouting matches and derogatory name calling that is the staple of many so called pubs and bars. Many arguments start out in a good-natured way, but often turn sour and the fun soon ends. Avoid hanging around in bars, there are many more things in this life one can do than waste so much time on a pastime that brings no reward.

In both examples mentioned here the common element is loudness and aggressiveness. It is exactly the loudness and aggressiveness that is out of place or "uncommon" that is the red flag—the warning. They are not the normal, polite, gentle interactions people engage in during "normal" conversation in everyday life—people just don't go around being loud and aggressive whether in a bar, a mall, or anywhere else unless there is something wrong with the situation or wrong with themselves.

Also watch for people who don't seem to "fit" where they are—someone who may just seem to be standing (or sitting) in a place or in a way that interferes with the normal flow of foot traffic—they'll stand out almost as much as someone sitting in the middle of the road. This also applies to people whose car is parked in an area or in a driveway you know no one ever parks in. Walk around and avoid the area. If you are concerned, you should call the police. If everything checks out fine no harm will be done to anyone. But if there is mischief afoot the police are trained and prepared to end it quickly.

Teachers and parents may wish to add to this some of their own experiences so that students and their own children will know some of what to look for as danger signs.

TEN

DE-ESCALATION

Here we have another definition. De-escalation: To decrease in extent, volume, or scope.

I especially like the part of the definition that mentions the decrease in volume, because, as previously mentioned, volume is a good indicator of trouble or pending trouble. It seems loudness is the byproduct of anxiety, fear, frustration, anger, and self-righteousness. If you find yourself becoming loud you may wish to examine what it is that is triggering this behavior in you. You may find that when you tone down your voice others will tone down theirs as well. In this way, by toning down your voice, you help de-escalate a situation and quite possibly resolve an issue.

Use an apology to help tone down an escalating argument. It's not a sign of weakness to say, "I'm sorry, but I don't see it that way." If you are wrong you can say you are wrong. "I'm sorry, I was wrong. I thought . . . ." Clear up misunderstandings as soon as possible so that no one feels like they are being made a fool of. If you can see that the person does not want to be rational, end the conversation, make an excuse and leave. There is right and there is dead right. Depending on where and with whom you are dealing, you must know your limitations and recognize when a situation is going badly.

Also, there are times when ignoring someone is the answer; not everything someone says needs a response or a snappy comeback—situation comedies on television have a 'laugh track', but real life does not, and becoming flip may make an awkward situation worse. There may be times when turning a deaf ear is the de-escalation solution. There is seldom any need to get caught up in an ever growing war of words. Bullies like to use words to try to test a possible target for weakness, fear, or controllability. There may come a time when simply looking at a bully and not responding is the appropriate response.

Now, read this carefully: Since my students are trained in physical self-defense and have rehearsed many different scenarios and are self-confident, they will recognize many of the situations described in this book.

We have talked about them. We have practiced them. And many have actually had to use some of the ideas or techniques contained herein. One of the techniques we use to discourage a bully's taunts or threats is the gentle smile. That's it—a smile. Students say nothing. The smile has a disconcerting effect on those who expect a negative response. It throws them off balance. Students have told me the bully simply went away. This, too, is de-escalation. If they give up and move on, then we have won through the principle of non-violence. If they don't give up, then the students can take whatever appropriate measures they feel they need to take to convince the bully to stop or to move on. The point I wish to make here is that through training, with permission, and understanding of what is going on around them, students can move from one type of self-defense to another. This takes time, a little patience, and practice.

Eleven

A WORD ABOUT STRANGERS

We warn our children about strangers, yet we send our children out among them every day. We warn them not to talk to strangers, but every day they are doing exactly that—talking to strangers and going places with them. We tell our children to avoid any adult who asks for their help finding a lost puppy—as if all strangers only follow one script to trick children. But children are fooled in many and often complicated ways. In short, we try very hard to protect children from abuse or abduction, but all too often we fail to tell them who or what a stranger is, because "stranger" is a concept, not a description.

When it comes to talking to our children about strangers we must remember to tell them "everyone is a stranger". The bus driver, for example, is a stranger; he is responsible for driving the bus, he is not supposed to ask any child to unbutton an article of clothing. Their classroom teacher is responsible for teaching lessons in the classroom, and is not supposed to take a child into the bathroom and touch parts of his or her body. We must let children know that everyone has a job or position in life and that people coming in and out of their lives cannot do or say things that are not in keeping with that position.

Here is a little experiment parents can do with their children in a public place and martial arts teachers can do in the studio: ask the children if there is or are strangers in the room. I have yet to receive a correct answer, and I am often met with complete silence as the children look at me and at each other—perhaps looking for something "strange". At this point I let them off the hook and point out the fact that everyone around us is a stranger, not only to us, but to each other. I tell them that unless people are very close family members we cannot tell if they are good or bad, because people can be either good or bad at any given time—it's only human nature. I tell my students, much to their surprise, that I am a stranger because they only know me as a teacher in the studio and that I'm not directly responsible for their everyday health, protection, shelter and wellbeing.

As mentioned, people in authority can control others, but they must do so only to a point they should not cross.

40

But this also begs a question of parental authority or the authority granted by parents to other family members, even to estranged parents. For our intent and purpose the use of the term "stranger" will not include immediate family members. This question is by far the hardest to answer because it really doesn't come under the banner of stranger abduction, but is related to abduction nonetheless. This type of abduction or abuse is a betrayal of trust within the family as well as a betrayal of the child's trust. The problem of abduction within the family can be mitigated by a greater degree of vigilance by the custodial parent, especially during times of breakup or divorce—the most commonly reported type of abduction. There is no substitute for constant vigilance and for keeping the children as close as possible at all times.

All this being said, it is not my intention, and it should not be your intention, as well, to cause undo fear in children of people around them—what a terrible world this would be—but to simply make children aware—in a caring way—that not everyone loves us or them, or is even our friend. If approached with love and kindness, children can be taught to be safe, or at least safer, by kind advice about strangers.

TWELVE

WOMEN and SELF-DEFENSE

Many women take self-defense classes because they want to know there is "something" they can do on their own behalf if they are attacked, for example, by someone while they are out jogging or loading groceries in their car after shopping. Self-defense seminars for women—periodically held by fire or police departments or local martial arts schools—not only include physical techniques to use if grabbed or attacked, but also try to impart the need for constant awareness that is such a big part of the self-protection equation. The classes are "women only", and seminars are generally kept light and casual and everyone goes home ready for anything, or so it is hoped.

Women at these self-defense seminars are learning the exact same tips, tricks, and techniques everyone else is learning in mixed-gender/ mixed age studios, and it makes one wonder why special classes for women are needed at all. Surely they can't be learning to defend themselves exclusively against other women. If women are to defend themselves against men, then it would be helpful to have an assortment of shapes and sizes of men on hand to make the training as real as possible. But as it is, there is usually one man covered from head to toe in foam padding upon whom women are encouraged to punch, kick, and scream at; a feel-good moment, to be sure, but far from realistic.

That's not to say all self-defense classes are of the feel good variety. It's just that too much of the realism is missing from the training. I propose we consider the following in women's self-defense training: men and women in regular street clothes—and with their shoes on—training and sparring together, as well as practicing chokes, grabs, pushing and pulling on each other while being verbally assaulted (sound familiar?); men attempting to control and command women physically and mentally. In short, a much more realistic and dynamic learning atmosphere than mere punching a foam-padded man can give; it becomes an exercise that helps teach women to stand up to men attempting to bully or attack them. If the training is not realistic then there is little point in wasting time and money—and maybe our future well being—learning something which has little value in the real world.

We must all face the reality that self-defense cannot be taught "after the fact" to deal with an event that has already happened—the time when many look for lessons—it can only demonstrate that there was something we could have done if only we knew it. The time for self-defense thoughts and lessons are always now before the need for self-protection and physical self-defense are upon us in the form of a stranger in a parking lot, for example, or an irate and belligerent spouse. Taking self-defense classes after an assault has happened may make us feel better, but it can't change what happened or the damage already done.

Learning self-defense will also better enable young girls and teens to recognize potential abusers and violent people—something that may save them much hardship and grief regarding domestic partnerships. When we come right down to it, stripped of financial and emotional attachments, what we have is someone we have made a conscious decision to share our personal space with—a stranger or near-stranger. Learning self-defense—and the attendant self-confidence and self-esteem that often results from such training—better prepares young girls to be confident in their abilities to care for themselves than those with no training at all—after all, it would be a rare person who would not consider their own health and well-being if they knew they could be hurt by their intended victim. Learning self-defense gives women that fighting chance.

THIRTEEN

A GOOD PUNCH

Before we get into the dynamics of punching I would like to clear up a couple of recurring myths about martial arts—the beliefs that practitioner's hands need to be registered with authorities, and the often heard necessity of warning an attacker or opponent of your karate prowess. In more than twenty years of practice, and having met hundreds of martial artists, I have never met one that had to register any part of their anatomy with anyone, anywhere. The idea of having to register anyone's hands makes no sense whatsoever. Why not register feet, or elbows, or knees? There is nothing different with respect to a martial artist's finger, for example, and someone else's untrained finger—a finger in the eye is still a finger in the eye no matter who does it. No registration required.

You also do not need to warn your attacker, or potential opponent, antagonist, drunk, or neighborhood bully of any skill you possess. Not only would it give them advance warning that they are dealing with a trained person, it could give someone the idea to bring friends or weapons to any confrontation with you—maybe even prepare an ambush. No warnings required. Don't do it—not even to try to impress people—it could easily backfire.

More immediate and important is the care needed while training to protect our hands from any damage, whether it is sprained wrists, abrasions, or broken fingers. One way to avoid possible problems that can result from training is to learn to punch correctly.

Children, especially those under the age of thirteen, should not be encouraged to punch any hard, or very dense, surfaces. There are 'heavy bags' that are too dense for young hands to punch without compromising safety. Youngster's bones have not yet fully formed, as has bone structures in adults, and they are much more susceptible to injury than is an adult. That is not to say that they should not strike at all. They could, perhaps, strike something similar to the vinyl-covered foam pads or hand mitts available at martial arts studios, or from boxing and kickboxing catalogues. The point is to teach any novice to punch on a softer surface than an experienced person would use. But proper punching does need to be taught and supervised so that students understand the techniques involved.

In striking with the fist, it is important to keep the wrist straight in relation to the forearm. Keeping the back of the fist in a straight line with the forearm will serve two purposes.

First, it will reduce the chance of injury—whether sprain, fracture, or dislocation of the wrist bones (known as carpals).

Second, the proper fist position allows for a greater transfer of force to the intended target.

When striking with the fist it is important to keep both feet in contact with the ground, yet keeping the body's weight on the balls of the feet by taking weight off of the heels ever so slightly. This is necessary in order to help us to slightly pivot our body when we deliver the strike—the more twist, or torque, we generate, the more powerful the strike will be. For example, if you were to punch with your left hand you would want to rotate your left hip ever so slightly forward a micro-second before you actually punch. Likewise, if you were to punch with the right hand, you would ever so slightly rotate your right hip forward a micro-second before the punch is executed for maximum effect. A little practice is all it takes to learn to punch correctly. If you have ever watched boxers in action you have seen what has been described herein—you just may not have noticed it at the time.

Parents can help train youngsters in the art of punching by holding their own palm, or palms, out so that the child has a target on which to focus and punch. The idea is not to have them demonstrate how hard they can hit—that they will do willingly. Our goal is simply to teach youngsters to focus and lightly strike as if working toward better eye and hand coordination. Parents should try not to be too critical of a novice's punching power—it will come with repetition—don't forget, you were once young and inexperienced too. Offering encouraging feedback will go a long way to effective learning. And parents, let's not forget that you too need to protect your hands. Keep your fingers together and your thumbs tucked tightly to the side of the index finger so as not to suffer your own sprains and strains due to young punches gone astray from your targeted palm.

Also, an old couch cushion can serve as an ideal shield on which to practice. As a matter of fact, a couch cushion can serve a multitude of purposes other than punching—kicking can also be practiced with the cushion as well.

Many martial arts schools advocate using the first two knuckles of the fist when punching. I do not agree with them for reasons I have already discussed. To turn the fist slightly outward in order to better expose the first two knuckles is to place the fist in an unnatural position—something that can lead to a dislocation, or break. Also, I don't believe we would be thinking of just how well our knuckles are exposed during an immediate self-defense situation.

The best fist, in my experience, is one in which the fist is kept on the same plane—straight with the forearm—and to punch with the entire fist. If done in the manner described, the middle knuckle will lead the way naturally, and since the middle knuckle is most forward it will impart a tremendous force at the point of impact. No cocked fist, no unnatural position—just power.

In summary, the best fist and best punch is one which includes a straight fist, incorporates the whole body behind the punch, and is not unnaturally cocked in favor of any particular pair of knuckles.

FOURTEEN

OF PALMS AND SLAPS

Balling the hands to make a fist is one of the first things many parents teach their children, especially when giving instructions on how to "punch him on the nose!", or "hit him back!" Good intentions, to be sure, but not the only option available. In this chapter we'll examine an alternate use of the hands for self-defense—palms and slaps—not only because they are applied differently than punches, but because they can belie and conceal not only their true power, but can also conceal what others believe they see happening.

Let's consider a scenario in which punching is used for self-defense. In the following example we will assume two people were fighting, and that there were witnesses to the fight.

In any group setting people will see different things happening depending on where they are standing in relation to others in the same setting even though they may be no more that a few feet from each other. What most will agree on—if they were looking in the same direction—is that there was a fight and that two individuals were punching each other. In other words, witnesses would say that BOTH were, in fact, punching each other as mutual combatants. Both had balled fists, an exchange had taken place, and we don't know who was the attacker and who was defending himself. Like a latecomer to a car accident, we ask what happened and get varying answers. One person may believe that one of the combatants was the aggressor, and someone else thought it was the other way round. No initial clear distinction is made.

Let's change the dynamics of the preceding example. The fight now has one of the combatants using his fists and the other has his hands up and open—palms forward and at shoulder height—in what looks like a placating manner, and may even look to some observers as if he has surrendered.

Witnesses can now clearly see who they believe is the aggressor and who the defender is—something that can be very useful if one should ever have to defend himself in court, as a result, perhaps, for being arrested for having to defend himself on the street.

The person who uses his fists does not necessarily stand a greater chance to win in a confrontation than does one who uses his palms. Palms can deliver a strike many times more powerful than a punch and with less chance of damage to the hands. A simple experiment will show this to be true.

To experience just how powerful a palm strike can be I suggest one stand close to a wall—a dense or hard surface, even a pine board will do—and with balled fist, start gently striking the chosen surface. It will not take too long to conclude that while you can build up a certain amount of power in your punch you can't punch any harder without much pain to yourself.

Now try the experiment with the heel of your palm. It doesn't take long to realize that you can strike with so much more force with so little effect on your hands.

Palms give one the ability to strike quite hard and yet not seem to be doing so. Training to strike with the palms is not complicated; all one needs is something like an overstuffed laundry-bag, or a couch cushion, to practice on.

Practice striking, pushing, and a combination of strikes and pushes to get the feel of the strike, and to develop the body mechanics needed effectively use palms in self-defense.

Children seem to respond very well to palm techniques, and like to practice as if it were a game. I believe that as a long as they are learning something useful, why not have a little fun along the way?

As far as open-hand techniques are concerned, there are few that can compare with the power of a well executed and well timed slap. I'm not talking about daytime television soap opera, Jane hates John slaps—I'm talking about a slap that uses the whole hand against the whole side of someone's head. This type of slap is quite capable of knocking someone down, and may even cause one to be knocked out or concussed.

This particular strike goes by various names depending on who is being taught the technique. It has been called a "combat slap" by teachers of military combatives courses. It has been called the "bouncer slap" by those working some of the larger and more rowdy night clubs. And I call it the "bully slap" when I'm speaking and teaching self-defense to youngsters. It would follow logically that if one were to teach self-defense to women it could be called the "mugger slap." Call it what you will, as long as you do it correctly.

The power of this technique comes from the use of the whole body in its execution. For, example, if you were to slap with your right hand you would want to keep the right hand down and close to your thigh—try not to look too obvious of your intention even during practice—until you are ready to unleash the strike. The right hand will travel in as continuous an arch as possible to the intended target. It's not a two-step action, but rather only one movement that includes the whole body in its execution. And the slap, or rather, the force of the slap, once it connects with the target should be such that the there is no choice for the attacker to go anywhere but down. In other words, for this, or any, technique to work, we must commit ourselves—especially if our lives depend on it.

Open-hand techniques are—for whatever reason—looked upon more favorably by society, and judges in a court of law, presumably because it is thought to cause less damage that a balled up fist. I guess as long as it doesn't resemble the all too familiar "karate chop," or look like someone has had special training that it somehow is more forgivable to use in self-defense. As such I have included them here because of the ease with which they can be learned and the power that can be delivered in time of need.

As in all things new, we must not only practice slowly, but we must practice with determination in order to become proficient—what we can do slowly and well, we can do quickly and well, too. We must always remember what these techniques are used for—to stop a determined effort to hurt us—and we must temper our response to what is actually happening. It would not do anyone any good to be struck in any manner herein described for trivial issues—such as name calling, or a simple misunderstanding over a toy, or an argument over a parking space—as you too could be held to answer for your actions to a policeman or a judge. Learn, teach, and practice with care.

FIFTEEN

A Few Tips and Talking Points

I would like to include in our conversation some observations and personal beliefs. In the end it is my hope that you will keep the conversation going with your teachers, parents, and students. The field of self-defense and self-protection is immense and no one can cover everything in one book, but we can get to the essence of what real training should accomplish and start a dialogue that can be continued in the schools and homes of all who are interested in martial arts and self-preservation. It is precisely because there are people who think kindness is a weakness, and gentleness an excuse to abuse someone that we must learn to stand up for ourselves and for those who cannot stand up for themselves. I hope your conversations are many.

Boxing for Boys and Girls

I advocate we teach all young people—boys as well as girls—the fundaments of boxing. By practicing boxing children would learn that they can't always win (or lose) because a win (or lose) today is no guarantee of the same outcome tomorrow. It places all children at an equal advantage, and when everyone has the same advantage people tend to be a bit more polite toward one another. I have yet to meet, or hear of, a student of martial arts or boxing who turned out to be a bully.

An argument could be made for an increase of the use of weapons for self-defense. I would argue that way too many weapons are used in assaults and self-defense now! Children, and adults, without training resort to weapons because they don't know there are other ways to defend themselves that do not include the use of a weapon. Children, too, often bring weapons to school to deal with bullies because their fear of being hit is so great or their frustration unbearable. Perhaps boxing skills can help reduce the need for weapons or the fear of being struck.

Simple safety measures relating to cars

An easy and free way to protect yourself and your valuables when riding in your car is to lock the doors immediately when you get it—that includes the driver's side door, as well. Locking the doors will prevent someone opening the door to steal your possessions or take your car. It is one of the easiest things we can do—along with buckling our seat-belts—to help insure our safety. Lock yourself in.

Don't leave valuables in plain sight even in a locked car. Windows can easily be broken causing additional loss and expensive repairs. Hide everything: cameras, loose change, even broken items you know have no value, thieves don't know if the items a broken or not. Put your possessions in the trunk of you vehicle—it is the most secure place because everything is out of sight. But remember to be as discrete as possible when packing things in the trunk. We don't want to advertise what we're doing because even trunks can get broken into. Be discrete!

Another awareness reminder

It is prudent to look behind you from time to time when doing any outside activity. Just watch the little birds as they feed—their heads are always bobbing up and down as they constantly check their environment. We don't have to be as cautious as the birds, perhaps, but it is important to know if we are being followed. Being "followed" and being "stalked" is to be followed by bad news no matter what we call it. If you feel uncomfortable with someone walking behind you— maybe they are a bit closer than you would like—simply stop as if you have just remembered something important and need a second to think about it. In doing so, you can maneuver yourself to let the person pass by, change your direction, or to defend if necessary. People have been attacked because they have ignored their uneasy feeling about someone behind them but felt it would be rude to look back to check. It's not paranoia. Trust your instincts.

You are that book-cover

They say, "Don't judge a book by its cover," but often the cover is all we get to look at in order to make a decision. How someone dresses—including you—is telling society who we are. People do make judgments based on what they see, and it does cause people to judge us—like it or not. I'm not talking about "civil rights" or "freedom of expression and freedom of speech"; I'm talking about people reading something in what we wear that will motivate them to approach or abuse us, or even avoid us. I'm talking about safety. If you dress like a "gangster", don't be surprised if people avoid you or treat you poorly—not too many gangsters are liked or respected. If you dress like a hooker, don't be offended or surprised if people talk down to you or talk in "fresh" or offensive ways. For all they know you may be advertising your services. How we look and how we present ourselves to others does have an effect upon how people treat us—ask any job applicant if this is not so.

Your own "bodyguard"

You really are your own bodyguard.

It's a given that society cannot afford to pay a policeman to walk with us all day every day. We have to learn to do many things for ourselves—such as dealing with bullies. From the moment we rise from our bed to the time we climb back in, we have to care for ourselves in myriad ways: brushing our teeth to protect from tooth decay, buckling our seat-belts to protect us in an accident, etc. That same logic applies when we go anywhere at any time. If we can understand the need to be aware of our surroundings and the people in it, we in fact become our own bodyguards—it would be so much more difficult to harm us or catch us unaware.

A note to teachers

Martial arts teachers and experts take note: Ever since we started teaching "realistic" techniques and scenarios in our class our retention rate vastly improved. Students and parents are pleased to see their children working in street clothes and shoes learning about self-protection in the real world. This is not to say we are not providing a good service "now", it simply means we can do much better without much effort or expense.

* Don't be there *

Avoidance is always easier than having to fight your way out of problems with others. If your instincts tell you that something is wrong, something probably is. Leaving the scene of a potential fight or dangerous situation or "dare" could save your life.

* Knowledge really is power *

Because self-defense is more than being able to kick or punch, we need to be able to defend ourselves in every environment because people can try to take advantage of us in situations not related to punching or kicking. Develop a healthy curiosity about how finances, politics, automobiles, and many things in our lives work. Knowledge will help keep us from being cheated. Stay in school.

* Stay in shape *

Try to stay in good physical shape or get into shape so as to be better able to defend yourself if you have to. You don't need to be in body-builder shape or loose mountains of weight, but you should have a modest exercise program.

* Saying "no" *

It is very rare for someone you do not know to offer you drugs or alcohol. The person most likely to do that is someone you know and who feels comfortable enough with you to suggest one or the other. Many times the person with influence is someone like a friend or cousin—maybe an older sibling—who will offer things to drink or take. Having a response that may keep such offers away can be, "I can't touch that stuff because I have a bad heart (or whatever you have rehearsed)." In this way you can distance yourself from having to take anything that can hurt you. Think of, and practice, a response before you need one.

Acknowledgements and Conclusion

I would like to thank Jeanne Raphael for giving me the encouragement to put my thoughts into words, and for helping me develop some of the thoughts herein with many questions and feed-back. Thanks are also due my sister Irene Mello, and my niece Raven Mello, for proof reading this work and offering their suggestions on making it better. There are a large number of people, too large, in fact, to be listed here that are due their thanks, as well. To all my teachers throughout my lifetime who have taught me so much about martial arts and life, I offer my thanks. To all my students who have proved to me that the theories work, I offer my thanks as well.

I conclude here as I have started—by saying that everything is self-defense. We would not like this world of ours to be violent, but it is, sometimes. Even good people have bad things happen to them. I hope you take away a few ideas and can make them work for yourself, your child, or your student. Perhaps if we really can help one life breathe easier because we have lived we will have succeeded.

I wish everyone a safe, happy and healthy life. I sincerely hope you find this little book helpful.

Peace,
Edward DeMedeiros, Master